The Mind, The Motion

STEPHANIE WATSON

Stephanie Watson can be reached as follows:
Email: fit2live.ca@gmail.com
Website: fit2live.ca
Instagram: @fit2live.ca

Published by Prominence Publishing www.prominencepublishing.com

ISBN: 978-1-988925-17-2
First Edition: January 2018

ACKNOWLEDGEMENTS

Thank you to those who made this book possible.

First, I'd like to thank my mom Cathy for her endless support.

I'd like to thank Matt for his confidence in me and for motivating me to continue writing.

I'd also like to thank Dan Cunningham and Brittany Grieve for editing and helping me create the finished product.

Finally, I'd like to thank my good friend Reena for making me feel like this book is going to help others.

TABLE OF CONTENTS

INTRODUCTION

Growing up, my ideal body image has always been to have a fit and toned figure. That is more easily achieved through a rigid structure, but I'm a spontaneous person and I don't think rigid structures are necessarily healthy. My view of *healthy* is living a lifestyle that frees one from being obsessed by body image, instead forming habits that foster confidence and self control over one's health.

This perspective drove me to doing extensive research and starting my company Fit2Live Fitness. My goal is to use my experience and education to provide guidance to any reader who has struggled with weight control and body image.

The Mind, The Motion shares what I believe is needed both mentally and physically to succeed. The first three chapters focus on three elements - the mind, nutrition, and exercise. The fourth chapter ties these elements together in an example of a 20 day program.

CHAPTER 1

MINDSET

A healthy mental state plays a critical part in weight control. Weight represents multiple things - possible water retention, dehydration, fat loss, and muscle gain. Although measuring weight by a scale can be very satisfying when the scale goes down, it can also be very discouraging when it doesn't. There are many other ways to measure progress that are arguably much more accurate.

<u>Alternate Ways to Measure Progress</u>

1. Pictures
   - Taken at the same time of day, wearing the same thing, improves accuracy.
2. Measurements
   - The waist reflects the fat in one's organ region, known as visceral fat. This measurement is very telling of an overall increase or decrease in body fat as well as possible bloating/water retention.
   - With a measuring tape, stand upright and breathe out (don't suck in). Tip left, then tip right. This is where the tape should sit for measuring.
3. Performance
   - running faster
   - more endurance
   - lifting heavier
4. How clothes fit
5. Energy and mood
   - increased energy
   - less napping

- better sleeps
- mental clarity
- elevated mood

It's important to feel confident and take pride in our bodies, but weight control should first and foremost be for health. This can be difficult because society puts so much emphasis on how we look. The pressure we put on ourselves to meet these high standards has contributed to binge eating being one of the most common eating disorders in the United States.

The reality is our appearance plays a very small role in our health. Positivity - that is, our attitude and ability to see good in ourselves - that brings a significant difference. Positivity creates motivation which leads to consistency in our actions.

Being consistent in our actions and positive in our outlook leads to progress and goal achievement. These positive experiences create satisfaction rather than a constant desire for change.

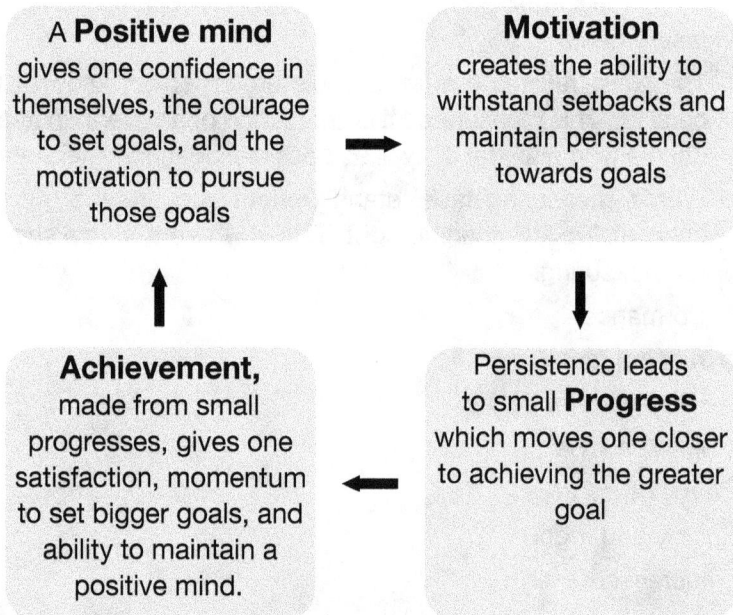

A **Positive mind**
gives one confidence in themselves, the courage to set goals, and the motivation to pursue those goals

➡️

Motivation
creates the ability to withstand setbacks and maintain persistence towards goals

⬆️

Achievement,
made from small progresses, gives one satisfaction, momentum to set bigger goals, and ability to maintain a positive mind.

⬅️

Persistence leads to small **Progress** which moves one closer to achieving the greater goal

⬇️

By creating a healthy mind, physical appearance naturally becomes secondary. Weight control becomes a challenge rather than a reflection of self worth. Positivity makes the challenge more enjoyable and in turn, more achievable.

Mindset Review

1. Name four things that weight represents?

   1._____   3._____

   2._____   4._____

2. Outside of using a weigh scale, name five other ways to measure progress?

   1._____   4._____

   2._____   5._____

   3._____

3. _____ plays a larger role in our in health than _____ does.

4. Progress and goal achievement come from being _____ in our actions and _____ in our outlook.

CHAPTER 2

NUTRITION

A strong grasp of nutrition will have a substantial impact on controlling weight. Knowledge of, and forming habits of healthy eating will provide long term, sustainable results.

Calories, Metabolism and Hydration

Calories are units of energy our bodies need to survive. If we consume more calories than we expend, the excess are stored as fat for future use. If we expend more calories than we consume, the body is going to break down fat and muscle simultaneously for energy in order to function.

Metabolism is how quickly the body uses calories. A person with a *fast* metabolism uses more calories than a person with a *slow* metabolism. If one is trying to lose weight, one will want to either increase metabolic rate; decrease caloric consumption; or increase caloric expenditure. The challenge with weight loss, is that when less calories are consumed, metabolism is slowed. This happens because the body has a natural preference to remain stable. When metabolism is slowed, less calories are needed by the body and weight loss stops (or plateaus).

This is why crash dieting does not work. Extremely low calorie diets for extended periods of time aren't enjoyable, healthy, or realistic.

Weight loss should be gradual because the body becomes accustomed to change. Small changes can be built upon and are more easily sustained than dramatic changes. Gradual weight loss helps prevent rebounding to one's starting point. Think of a fast weight loss program as going up a hill, and a gradual program as going up a set of stairs. The only spots on a hill where there is stability is at the top and at the bottom. On a flight of stairs there is stability at each step.

That is where *reverse dieting* plays an important role. Reverse dieting is the process of slowly increasing daily calorie consumption in order to allow the metabolism time to speed up. If one continues to exercise during this time, more muscle can be gained, contributing to a faster metabolism as well.

Hydration The benefits and importance of hydration are endless regarding weight control. Staying hydrated helps prevent the body from saying "I'm hungry" when it actually isn't. This is partially due to the fact that the body receives water and food at the same point - the stomach. Therefore, it's going to feel very similar when the body is signaling thirst or hunger.

Hydration also speeds up the body's metabolism, helps with food breakdown, keeps digestive regularity, and reduces fatigue. Water is so crucial to bodily health and it's the easiest part to get right. The focus is consumption rather than restriction. Three to four liters of water a day is a great target to ensure hydration.

MacroNutrients and MicroNutrients

MacroNutrients are nutrients that the body needs in large amounts. There are three of them - carbohydrates, proteins, and fats.

Carbohydrates are the body's preferred energy source and are stored in the liver and muscles where they are readily available for short term energy. Excess carbohydrates are kept as fat. Each gram of carbohydrate is four calories of energy.

Carbohydrates high in fibre can be super helpful with weight control, as they keep one regular, give one the feeling of being full, and stabilize blood sugars. There are two types of fibre - soluble and insoluble. Soluble fibre absorbs water and works like a sponge in the digestive tract. Insoluble fiber does not absorb water, and works like a broom to sweep everything along the digestive tract.

High Fibrous Carbohydrates	Low Fibrous Carbohydrates
fruits	candy
vegetables	white pasta
whole grain bread and wraps	white bread
oats	sugary cereal
legumes	gatorade
seeds	pop
etc.	pastries
	etc.

Carbohydrates low in fibre tend to be high in sugar which can be detrimental to weight control for two reasons:

1. INSULIN RESISTANCE. Insulin is a hormone whose job is to notify cells in the body to let sugar in. Cells need sugar for energy. When one chooses high sugar options, there is an increase in the amount of insulin in their body. Too much insulin causes cells to begin resisting insulin's instruction to utilize the sugar. This is known as insulin resistance and can lead to many health issues such as diabetes.

2. ADDICTION. Sugar is extremely addictive. The more one feeds an addiction, the stronger it becomes. The constant desire for more sugar makes keeping calories under control very difficult.

All carbohydrates - fruit, grains, vegetables, candy - are converted to glucose eventually. However the more fibrous and complex options one consumes, the more full they will be and the more vitamins and minerals they will consume. Therefore the likelihood of overconsumption will decrease.

Protein is used for the formation of the brain, nervous system, blood, muscles, skin and hair. It assists in the transportation of nutrients and antibodies, and accelerates chemical reactions in the body. Partly because it takes the most energy for the body to break down, protein also aids in a lean body composition. Each gram of protein is four calories of energy.

Protein low in saturated fat is typically lower in calories as well.

Low Saturated Fat Protein	High Saturated Fat Protein
Chicken breast	chicken wings
turkey breast	ribs
shellfish	chicken skin
white fish	fatty red meat
egg whites	sugary, high calorie protein drinks
lean cuts of red meat	etc.
low-fat greek yogurt	
wild salmon	
low fat protein drinks	
etc.	

Fat is used for insulation, cell structure, vitamin absorption, and hormone production. Each gram of fat has 9 calories of energy.

Although fats are essential to health, keep in mind their high caloric value. Fats low in nutritional value should be eaten minimally. Omega 3, 6 and 9 are all healthy fats (see below). The average North American obtains 6 and 9 readily through the foods we eat, however, we typically struggle to get enough Omega 3. Omega 3 aids in protecting and maintaining a healthy heart, as well as brain health and function. For these reasons, the addition of an Omega 3 supplement every morning may be beneficial.

Healthy Fats	Unhealthy Fats
avocado	high fatty red meats
nuts	poultry skin
cheese	chips
dark chocolate	deep fried foods
whole eggs	pastries
coconut	cookies
nut oils	etc.
seeds	
fatty fish	
butter	
omega 3 supplementation	
etc.	

Each macronutrient has a very important purpose in relation to bodily function and health. By making healthy choices it's much easier to feed the body the nutrition it needs without a surplus of calories.

There is more to weight control than counting calories and macronutrients. Because, overall health should be the main focus, and that isn't fully achieved without also consuming what our bodies need in small amounts - micronutrients.

Micronutrients are composed of vitamins and minerals. Although they are only needed in small amounts, they play an important role in good health.

There are thirteen vitamins required by the human body. Their role includes releasing energy from carbohydrates, fats & proteins; building tissues, bone and teeth; developing cells; and strengthening the nervous system. Nine of the thirteen vitamins are water soluble (they flush out of the body through the urine) which means they must be ingested every day.

Like vitamins, minerals are also critical for survival. Amongst other things, they create a balanced pH in the body. Minerals also balance bodily fluids and help the body resist stress and disease.

Think of the body as an apple - once exposed to oxygen, the apple will brown and rot very quickly. Vitamins and minerals have antioxidizing effects that act like the skin of an apple, decelerating this process.

Unhealthy Choices

Processed Food vs. Whole Foods. The more energy the body uses in digesting food, the better it is for weight control. Processing food can create a readily absorbable product; thus, the body doesn't expend as much energy digesting it.

There can also be many chemicals and by-products in processed foods that negatively affect digestive health and a lack of nutrients that reduce energy levels. Finally, processed foods are commonly higher in sugar which leads to an addictive nature and salt which leads to water retention.

Unhealthy Choices Although unhealthy choices (eg. fast food, soda, candy etc) aren't encouraged, they are part of life for most people. It is important to learn how to incorporate unhealthy choices in a way that isn't detrimental to one's goals.

Finding moderation is much healthier than to label things as bad or off limits. This labelling can increase their temptation and the damage done when one finally relents is often more harmful to the body and mental state as well. Practices such as committing to two bites then deciding if further indulgence is necessary may be helpful.

Alcohol beverages are primarily fermented sugar from grains and fruits and have seven calories of energy per gram. In large quantities it can be very harmful to physical and mental health - it increases lethargy; the likelihood of missing workouts and making unhealthy food choices. It also increases chances of sickness, depression, and other mental and physical diseases.

If choosing to drink alcohol while trying to control weight, the amount of calories absorbed through that consumption should be kept to a minimum because these empty calories are replacing nutrient dense calories absorbed from carbohydrates, fats, and/or protein. Clear spirits (vodka, gin, tequila, rum) with soda or water have around 65 calories per single ounce compared to a nine ounce glass of wine at about 180 calories.   Increasing water intake while drinking alcohol also keeps the body hydrated and slows the pace of consumption.

Willpower Any time one resists a craving, willpower is used. Willpower is a limited resource so the key is to preserve as much of it as possible. Nourishing the body with the right nutrition, getting adequate rest, and finding enjoyable healthy habits are three ways to preserve and replenish this valuable resource.

Cheat Meals and the need for them is an individual preference. Many find satisfaction in one cheat meal per week and find it is both physically and mentally beneficial for weight control. Bingeing during cheat meals, constantly thinking about the next one, or participating frequently in unplanned cheating, indicates a problem. If weight control is the goal, a consistent diet is ideal.

Supplementation

Supplementation is a convenient and effective way to improve overall health. High quality brands base their products off of the latest scientific research, maintain high quality control, and are easily absorbed by the body.

Multi-Vitamins can improve health. The risk of contracting many diseases such as cancer, heart attacks, bone loss, stroke, etc. can be reduced by consuming the right nutrients. It is very challenging to get all our needed nutrients through the food we eat alone.

Powdered Greens are fruits, vegetables, algae and grasses concentrated into powdered form. Amongst other things, they are designed to increase energy, boost metabolism, improve digestion, and act as anti-inflammatories.

Omega 3, commonly taken as fish oil, is linked to many health benefits including heart and brain protection, function, and overall health.

Whey Protein is derived from milk traditionally as a result of cheese production. It is a convenient and cost efficient way of increasing high quality protein intake.

Vegetarian Protein requires a combination of plants in order to create a complete protein. The most common blend is peas and rice. Vegetarian proteins are typically rich in vitamins and minerals, are high in antioxidants, and contain dietary fiber.

Supplementation and Weight Control

Supplements are found by many to be extremely helpful in achieving weight control. Others choose not to use supplements and still achieve desired results. It is up to the individual. There are many products that stimulate metabolism through ingredients like caffeine. Although they do work in the short term, the long term results aren't necessarily maintainable. Below are two well studied supplements that do not include stimulants and may safely be introduced to a daily routine.

L-Carnitine is found naturally in the body as well as in some of the food we eat. L-carnitine is suggested to be effective in breaking down fat to be utilized for energy. Research has shown it is most beneficial to take L-carnitine with carbohydrates for it to be effective. Dosage depends on the size and needs of the individual, and should be taken in proper dosages to avoid any negative side effects.

Conjugated Linoleic Acid (CLA): unlike L-carnitine, CLA is not made naturally by the body, instead it is ingested from foods such as dairy products and certain meat. CLA claims many health benefits, one being that it lowers insulin resistance. This increases fat utilization, rather than storage. Research suggests that one must take a minimum dose of 5g/day, preferably with food, for CLA to be effective.

Nutrition Review

1. What is a calorie?

_____

_____

2. What is a macronutrient?

_____

3. Name all three macronutrients and their functions:

   a. _____ :_____

   b. _____ : _____

   c. _____ : _____

4. Which macronutrient has the highest caloric value?

_____

5. What are three benefits of a diet high in fiber?

   1. _____

   2. _____

   3. _____

6. What are two risks of a diet high in sugar?

   1. _____

   2. _____

7. What is the benefit of protein options that are low in fat?

_____

8. Why is this beneficial?

_____

9. What are three healthy types of fat?

   1. _____

   2. _____

   3. _____

10. Name three benefits of hydration?

1. _____

2. _____

3. _____

11. Name five healthy and enjoyable carbohydrate, protein, and fat options all equivalent to 100 - 150 calories:

Carbohydrates	Protein	Fat
1.	1.	1.
2.	2.	2.
3.	3.	3.
4.	4.	4.
5.	5.	5.

CHAPTER 3

EXERCISE

'Exercise' is as simple as going for a brisk walk, or as difficult as running a marathon.

Exercise and Internal Health

Just as proper nutrition increases how efficiently the body functions, so does exercise. Keeping active enhances energy levels by delivering oxygen to all the cells of the body which is critical for their survival. Exercise of any kind enhances one's mood by releasing endorphins (the body's natural 'happy drug') as well as decreases the chance of mental diseases such as anxiety and depression. There is also a direct correlation between exercise and reduced risk of diseases such as obesity, diabetes, heart disease, and stroke. Finally, exercise is proven to enhance quality of sleep.

Exercise and Weight Control

Weight control comes more readily, and is more easily maintained with daily exercise. Not only does exercise increase the amount of daily calories burned, it can help build a faster metabolism. Three very effective exercises for weight control are high intensity interval training, exhaustive exercise and strength training.

High intensity interval training (HIIT) is undertaking periods of rapid movement and then periods of slower movement or rest. It is an effective way to burn a lot of calories quickly. The high intensity also increases growth hormone (GH) in the body. Growth hormone aids fat loss.

Exhaustive training is any activity which brings one to a point of exhaustion. It is another great way to burn a lot of calories. In addition, working out to exhaustion for 20-30 minutes has been shown to be one of the best ways for the body to produce glucagon, which is a fat burning hormone.

Strength training increases the amount of muscle cells in the body. Because muscle cells need more energy to survive than fat cells do, increased muscle mass increases the body's metabolic rate. Strength training also increases a fat burning hormone in the body known as testosterone.

The intensity or type of exercise isn't as important as the habit of exercise. Any type of exercise or activity is beneficial. Our bodies are made to move!

Exercise Review

1. How does keeping active enhance energy levels?

_____

_____

2. Exercise is linked to a decrease in mental diseases such as:

    a. _____

    b. _____

    c. _____

3. Exercise is linked to a decrease in physical diseases such as:

    a. _____

    b. _____

    c. _____

    d. _____

4. Exercise enhances quality of _____.

5. What are three types of exercise extremely effective for controlling weight?

    a. _____

    b. _____

    c. _____

CHAPTER 4

THE MIND, THE MOTION

As I said at the outset of this book, my purpose in writing it was to share what I've learned about the importance of positive thinking, good nutrition and exercise in achieving weight control. In this section, I'm combining these three elements in a 20 day balanced program. For each day, I offer a mental exercise to enhance positive thinking; an example meal plan of 400 calories/meal as a base for good nutrition; and a 40 minute regime to introduce daily exercise.

The brain is a very sophisticated muscle, but a muscle nonetheless. Therefore, to obtain its maximum potential, it should be exercised regularly. Consistently maintaining a positive outlook requires practise and conscious effort and should not be neglected. Just as it's easy to let weight get out of control, it's easy to let negativity take over the mind. Therefore, for each day, I've included a simple exercise to help the brain remain positive and plan for success.

Beside each day in the *progress calendar* at the end of this chapter, there are empty circles. Once the mental activity, a healthy breakfast, lunch or dinner is had, or a workout is completed, fill the circle in with a smiley face. This may seem insignificant, but the satisfaction of filling in the circles every day creates a positive response in the brain to carry on the bahavior. A little positive saying repeated as well as filling in the circle will enhance this response even further.

Food is meant to be enjoyed and is a large part of our lives and our culture. There are always new products, new restaurants, and new recipes to try. For each day, I've included ideas for breakfast, lunch, and dinner all equivalent to roughly 400 calories. While every individual needs a different caloric intake, three healthy 400 calorie meals a day provides a great base so that choices made outside of those meals are coming from a healthier more stable body. There is a list of snack ideas near the end of the book.

The majority of these recipes were made using a scale, and specific brands and weights of individual ingredients. The amount of calories per ingredient is shown in brackets on each chart. The reader should check the nutritional chart of the product he or she is using if he or she wishes to match exactly the amount of calories. (Note, roughly speaking a ½ cup is roughly equivalent to a cupped hand; a cup is roughly equivalent to a clenched fist; 3 oz is roughly the size of the palm of hand; and 1 tbsp is roughly the size of a thumb.)

The ideal meal is high in fiber, low in sugar, and balanced in the three macronutrients. This won't happen perfectly each time. For example, the reader may notice that some options I've offered are higher in sugar or carbohydrates and low in fiber. The important thing is that if one has a 'high sugar' day one day, the next day should be a 'low sugar' day. That's how a balanced diet is achieved. And balance is more important than obsessing over a meal plan.

The meal program included is based on a four day cycle. For the first three days, I provide meal ideas. For the fourth day, the reader creates their own. To save on cost and waste, use up perishable ingredients in the fridge, plan ahead and create a grocery list, or repeat any meal to minimize variety. Incorporate many vegetables, lean proteins and healthy fats. This will result in a larger meal and make controlling weight much easier. Any form of nutrition tracker may be used when creating meals.

The exercise program included, is based on a seven day cycle, in which almost all the major muscle groups are worked and the three styles of training (i.e. HIIT, exhaustive, and strength) beneficial for weight control are used. For successive weeks, different exercises which serve the same purpose are introduced so that the reader has some variety and can eventually choose the exercises that he or she prefers. Each seven day cycle includes an active rest day, during which a person should not become a couch potato, but rather engage in some form of enjoyable physical activity.

Listed beside some workouts are blank boxes. These are to be used to document what the reader did, questions that may arise or why a workout was missed. This is a great tool to measure progress and to push oneself past previous marks.

Starting weights for some exercises will vary from person to person. If the reader is unsure or nervous about injury, I recommend the guidance of a professional. Regardless, the reader should properly warm up before and stretch after all exercises.

Day	Date	Mental Activity	Healthy Breakfast	Healthy Lunch	Healthy Dinner	Exercise
1	_____	☐	☐	☐	☐	☐
2	_____	☐	☐	☐	☐	☐
3	_____	☐	☐	☐	☐	☐
4	_____	☐	☐	☐	☐	☐
5	_____	☐	☐	☐	☐	☐
6	_____	☐	☐	☐	☐	☐
7	_____	☐	☐	☐	☐	☐
8	_____	☐	☐	☐	☐	☐
9	_____	☐	☐	☐	☐	☐
10	_____	☐	☐	☐	☐	☐
11	_____	☐	☐	☐	☐	☐
12	_____	☐	☐	☐	☐	☐
13	_____	☐	☐	☐	☐	☐
14	_____	☐	☐	☐	☐	☐
15	_____	☐	☐	☐	☐	☐
16	_____	☐	☐	☐	☐	☐
17	_____	☐	☐	☐	☐	☐
18	_____	☐	☐	☐	☐	☐
19	_____	☐	☐	☐	☐	☐
20	_____	☐	☐	☐	☐	☐

Day 1

"The secret to change is to focus all of your energy,
not on fighting the old, but on building the new" —Socrates

Name 3 positive things that a healthier lifestyle will bring:

1. _____

2. _____

3. _____

Breakfast *Egg and Avocado Sandwich*

Ingredients

• 2 small slices whole grain bread (110) • 1 egg, over medium (72) • 3 slices turkey bacon (30 each: 90)	• ½ medium avocado, mashed (108) o dash of salt, pepper, garlic and small squeeze lemon • 1 roma tomato, sliced (18)

Nutrition Information

Carbohydrates: 31g Fat: 22g Protein: 19g	Calories: 398 Sugar: 4g Fiber: 10.5g

Lunch *Chicken stir-fry*

Ingredients

• 2oz cooked chicken breast (94) • 1 egg (72) • ½ avocado (100) • ½ medium red pepper (16) • spices: garlic, pepper, chili flakes, cumin, onion power, chili powder & parsley • lemon	• 1 small zucchini (26) • 10 spears asparagus (33) • ¼ cup chopped red onion (3) • 8 tbsp black bean and corn salsa (60)

Directions

1. *In a large pan or wok, add veggies to ½ cup of boiling water. Once water dissolves, put veggies onto a side plate. Add any type of seasonings or spices (recommend: garlic, pepper, chili flakes)*
2. *Cube chicken breast and add to medium frying pan over med-high heat. (sprayed with cooking oil)*
   a. *Add equal parts: cumin, chili flakes, parsley, onion powder, chili powder*
3. *Once chicken is cooked fully through, add egg and veggies and fry until egg is fully cooked.*
4. *Mash avocado with lemon, garlic, salt and pepper*
5. *Serve stir-fry and avocado with black bean and corn salsa.*

Nutrition Information

Carbohydrates: 29g	Calories: 402
Fat: 17g	Sugar: 12g
Protein: 30g	Fiber: 9.6g

Dinner *Shaken Taco Salad*

• ½ cup ground turkey, lean, raw (141)	• 5 grape tomatoes (18)
• ¼ cup medium salsa (26)	• ½ small avocado (80)
• 2 tbsp 0% greek yogurt (17)	• ½ medium bell pepper, sliced, any colour (15)
• ⅓ cup light shredded cheese (80)	
• ½ head iceberg lettuce (30)	• ½ tbsp lemon juice (2)

Directions

1. *Cook turkey on frying pan over med-high heat*
2. *Add salsa and simmer*
3. *Add lemon juice to yogurt and mix for sour cream.*
4. *Mash avocado*
5. *Optional *Add lemon, garlic, chili flakes to make guacamole*

6. *Add tomatoes, lettuce, peppers and cheese to sealable container*
7. *While still warm, add turkey and salsa, sour cream, and avocado. shake and pour onto plate or eat out of container.*

Nutrition Information

Carbohydrates: 24g	Calories: 410
Fat: 21g	Sugar 11g
Protein: 36g	Fiber: 9g

Exercise

Cardio: Timed Intervals

Minutes	Movement
(0-5)	Warm-up 5 minute jog
(5-35)	10 times through • 1 minute walk • 1 minute jog • 1 minute fast
(35-40)	Cool down 5 minute walk
	Stretch quads, hamstrings, calves, glute muscles
	Equipment needed treadmill or outdoor running space

Day 2

"Be stronger than your excuses" — Unknown

Write down 3 excuses/justifications for unhealthy eating and skipping exercise. Then, write a stronger rebuttal for each excuse.

1. _____
   _____
   _____
   _____
   _____

2. _____
   _____
   _____
   _____
   _____

3. _____
   _____
   _____
   _____
   _____

Breakfast *Mixed Berry Smoothie*

Ingredients

• 1 scoop vanilla protein powder (120)	• 1 tbsp Chia seeds (60)
• ½ cup 2% cottage cheese (110)	• ½ cup strawberries (39)
• 1 tbsp chopped pecan (39)	• ½ cup blueberries (32)

Nutrition Information

Carbohydrates: 32g	Calories: 400
Fat: 11g	Sugar: 17g
Protein: 44g	Fiber: 10g

Lunch *Turkey Sausage and Rosemary Squash*

Ingredients

• 2 cups butternut squash, cubed (126)	• 1 tbsp rosemary (2)
• 2 tsp butter (70)	• 2 turkey sausages (220)

Directions

1. *Preheat oven to 425 degrees fahrenheit*
2. *Line baking tray with aluminum foil*
3. *Toss cubed squash in melted butter*
4. *Place turkey sausage and cubed squash onto tray, spaced out in a single layer*
5. *Top squash with rosemary*
6. *Once squash is browning and sausage is fully cooked, remove*
7. *Slice turkey*

Nutrition Information

Carbohydrates: 43g Fat: 16g Protein: 31g	Calories: 416 Sugar: 12g Fiber: 6g

Dinner *Teriyaki Chicken Rice Bowl*

• 2.5 oz (just over ½ palm size) chicken breast, cooked (117)	• 5 small mushrooms, raw, white (11)
• ½ medium bell pepper, any color (16)	• 1 garlic clove (4)
• ½ tsp cumin (4)	• ⅓ small zucchini (8)
• ½ tsp parsley (1)	• 3 tbsp 0% plain greek yogurt (23)
• 1 tsp chili flakes	• 2 tbsp chopped walnuts (100)
• ½ cup brown rice, cooked (109)	• 1 tbsp teriyaki marinade (15)
• 2 tbsp red onion, finely sliced (2)	• 1/2 tbsp lime juice (2)

Directions

1. *Put rice in steamer and set aside.*
2. *Spicy yogurt: add lime juice, cumin, parsley and chili flakes to yogurt. mix and set aside.*
3. *Lightly spray pan over medium heat. cube and fry chicken until halfway cooked. add pepper, onion, mushroom and zucchini. add water if needed. cook until soft. add minced garlic, teriyaki marinade, and walnuts. simmer 3-5 minutes.*
4. *Serve over rice and top with yogurt*

Nutrition Information

Carbohydrates: 37g Fat: 14g Protein: 35g	Calories: 411 Sugar: 8g Fiber: 4g

Exercise

Strength Training : Major Back Muscles

Recommended warm-up: 5 minutes elliptical

Minutes	Movement	Notes	Notes
(0-5)	1. Straight-arm cable pressdowns 3 sets x15 repetitions (reps)		

(5-10)	2. Bent-over-bench single arm dumbbell
	   rows
	   3 sets X 15 reps per side		

(10-15)	3. Wide-grip pulldowns 3 sets X 15 reps		
(15-20)	4. Behind-head pulldowns 3 sets X 15 reps		
(20-25)	5. Seated cable pull-ins 3 sets X 15 reps		

(25-30)	6. Seated rows 3 sets X 15 reps		
(30-35)	7. Bent over barbell rows 3 sets X 15 reps		

(35-40)	8. Pull-ups to fail or assisted pull-ups
	    3 sets x to fail or
	    3 sets x 10 reps (assisted pull-ups)		

	Stretch back, neck, chest		

	Equipment needed
	    cable machine, dumbbells,
	    pulldown machine, row machine,
	    barbell, assisted pull up machine		

Day 3

"Know your strengths and take advantage of them" —Greg Norman

Identify 3 of your strengths and how you can utilize them to achieve your goals:

1. _____

2. _____

3. _____

Breakfast *Breakfast Quesadilla*

Ingredients

• flax tortilla (170)	• ¾ cup egg whites (90)
• ⅓ cup grated cheddar cheese (120)	• ¼ cup salsa (25)

Nutrition Information

Carbohydrates: 31g	Calories: 405
Fat: 14g	Sugar: 3g
Protein: 34g	Fiber: 6g

Lunch *Greek Yogurt Chicken*

Ingredients

• 1/2 cup 0% greek yogurt (67)	• 1 cup cubed cooked chicken breast, skinless (222)
• 1 tsp cider vinegar	• 1 cup chopped celery (19)
• 1 tsp poppy seeds (15)	• 1 tbsp dried cranberries (23)
• 1 tsp rosemary (1)	• 1 tbsp sliced almonds (48)
• salt and pepper, to taste	

Directions

1. *Mix vinegar, poppy seeds, yogurt, rosemary, salt and pepper*
   a. *let sit overnight if possible*
2. *Pour mixture over cooled chicken, celery, cranberries and almonds*

Nutrition Information

Carbohydrates: 16g	Calories: 394
Fat: 10g	Sugar: 11g
Protein: 60g	Fiber: 4g

Dinner *Roast Beef Dinner*

• 6 oz roast beef (210)	• ¼ cup sweet peas (25)
• ½ small-medium cauliflower head, steamed and blended (50)	• 1 large carrot, sliced and steamed (30)
• 2 tsp butter (68)	• 1 tbsp au jus gravy mix (20)

Nutrition Information

Carbohydrates: 30g	Calories: 402
Fat: 17g	Sugar: 13g
Protein: 40g	Fiber: 9g

Exercise

Strength Training: Lower Body

Recommended warm-up: 5 minutes stair climber

Minutes	Movement	Notes	Notes
(0-5)	1. Barbell hip thrust 3 sets x15 reps		
(5-10)	2. Barbell deadlifts 3 sets X 15 reps		
(10-15)	3. Abductors 3 sets X 15 reps		

(15-20)	4. Cable kickbacks 3 sets X 15 reps per side		
(20-25)	5. Curtsy lunge step-ups 3 sets X 10 reps per side		
(25-30)	6. Kettle bell swings 3 sets X 15 reps		
(30-35)	7. Side-lying leg raises 3 sets X 15 reps per side		
(35-40)	8. Hip hikes 3 sets x 15 reps per side		

	Stretch
	    hamstrings, glute muscles,
	    quads, lower back, calves		

	Equipment needed
	    barbell, abductor machine,
	    cable machine, bench,
	    kettlebell, dumbbells		

Day 4

> *"Self discipline begins with the mastery of your thoughts. If you
> control what you think, you control what you do"* —Unknown

Write down how good it feels the moment a workout is finished. The
next time you're procrastinating a workout, rather than thinking about
the dreaded activities, think of the feeling after it's done.

_____

_____

_____

_____

Breakfast _____

Ingredients

•	•
•	•
•	•
•	•

Directions

_____

_____

_____

Nutrition Information

Carbohydrates: _____g	Calories: _____
Fat: _____g	Sugar: _____g
Protein: _____g	Fiber: _____g

Lunch _____

Ingredients

•	•
•	•
•	•
•	•

Directions

_____

_____

_____

Nutrition Information

Carbohydrates: _____g	Calories: _____
Fat: _____g	Sugar: _____g
Protein: _____g	Fiber: _____g

Dinner _____

Ingredients

•	•
•	•
•	•
•	•

Directions

_____

_____

_____

Nutrition Information

Carbohydrates: _____g	Calories: _____
Fat: _____g	Sugar: _____g
Protein: _____g	Fiber: _____g

Exercise

Strength Training: Shoulders

Recommended warm-up: arm circles (30 forward and 30 backward)

Minutes	Motion		
(0-5)	1. Dumbbell shoulder press 3 sets x15 reps		
(5-10)	2. Arnold shoulder press 3 sets X 15 reps		
(10-15)	3. Lateral deltoid dumbbell raises 3 sets X 15 reps		
(15-20)	4. Dumbbell front deltoid raises 3 sets X 15 reps		
(20-25)	5.Seated leaned over rear deltoid raises 3 sets X 15 reps		
(25-30)	6.Crossed over rear deltoid cable pulls 3 sets X 15 reps per side		
(30-35)	7.Cable lateral deltoid raises 3 sets X 15 reps per side		
(35-40)	8.Resistance band rear delt pulses 3 sets x30 reps		
	Stretch neck and shoulders		
	Equipment needed dumbbells, barbell, cables		

Day 5

"Sometimes we miss a workout or eat something that isn't ideal, but if you had a flat tire on your car, would you get out and puncture the other three? Of course not! If you slip, shake it off, and do better the next try" —Jillian Michaels

Next time you fall off track, what 3 steps are going to get you moving back in the right direction?

1. _____

2. _____

3. _____

Breakfast *Blueberry Chia Smoothie*

Ingredients

• 1 scoop vanilla protein powder (115)	• 1 tbsp chia seeds (60)
• 1.5 cup unsweetened almond milk (45)	• 1 cup frozen unsweetened blueberries (80)
• ½ avocado (100)	• dash Cinnamon

Nutrition Information

Carbohydrates: 32g	Calories: 400
Fat: 17g	Sugar: 12g
Protein: 31g	Fiber: 14g

Lunch *Salmon, Kale and Blackberry Salad*

Ingredients

• 4oz farmed (or 5oz wild) salmon, baked, w/lemon & dill (245)	• 1 serving Sweet Kale Vegetable salad kit (140)
	• ⅓ cup blackberries (21)

Nutrition Information

Carbohydrates: 20g	Calories: 403
Fat: 23g	Sugar: 12g
Protein: 29g	Fiber: 5g

Dinner *Fish and Chips*

• 6oz cod, raw, fillet (120)	tartar sauce:
• 1 medium potato, white, skin (147)	• ¼ cup 0% greek yogurt (34)
• ½ + ¼ tbsp extra virgin olive oil (89)	• 1 tbsp parsley, fresh, chopped (2)
• ½ tbsp lemon zest (2)	• 1 tbsp capers, chopped (2)
• salt and pepper, to taste	• 1 lemon, juiced (10)

Directions

1. *Preheat oven to 400 degrees fahrenheit*
2. *Soak fish in ½ lemon juice, set aside*
3. *Slice potatoes into chips, toss in ½ tbsp olive oil and spread in an even layer onto baking tray. Bake until starting to golden*
   * about 30-40 minutes
4. *Put fish in glass casserole dish, brush with ¼ tbsp olive oil, salt and pepper*
   *bake 10-12 minutes. add ½ tbsp parsley and lemon zest for last 2-3 minutes of baking
5. *Tartar sauce: mix capers, remaining parsley and lemon juice into yogurt*

Nutrition Information

Carbohydrates: 40g	Calories: 405
Fat: 15g	Sugar: 5g
Protein: 31g	Fiber: 6g

Exercise

Cardio: Circuit training and *abs*

Minutes	Movement
(0-15)	1 minute each, 5 times through • Skipping • Jumping Jacks • Box jumps or Step-ups
(15-40)	1 minute each, 5 times through • Crunches • Kick downs with lift • Russian twists • Vacuums • Pulsing side plank (30s Left side, 30s Right side)
	Stretch abs, lower back, legs, calves
	Equipment needed skipping rope, medicine ball

Day 6

*"Stay committed to your decisions, but stay flexible
in your approach" —Anthony Robbins*

What is an obstacle you foresee coming in the next week that may
steer you from your goals? How can you improvise and overcome that
obstacle?

Obstacle: _____

Improvise: _____

Breakfast *Oats and Egg whites*

Ingredients

• ⅓ cup oats (measured dry) (120)
  dash cinnamon
• 1 tbsp natural peanut butter (90)
	• ¾ egg whites (90)
	• ½ medium avocado, mashed (100)
	  add lemon, hot sauce & garlic

Nutrition Information

Carbohydrates: 31g Fat: 18g Protein: 29g	Calories: 400 Sugar: 2g Fiber: 8g

Lunch *Buffalo Chicken Caesar Salad*

Ingredients

• 2 cups romaine lettuce (10) • 4 oz (palm size) chicken breast, baked and cubed (187) • ½ tbsp melted butter (51)	• 2 tbsp hot sauce (0) • 2 tbsp caesar dressing (80) • 3 tbsp light shredded parmesan cheese (68)

Directions

1. *Toss lettuce in dressing.*
2. *Toss chicken in melted butter and hot sauce.*
3. *Top with parmesan cheese.*

Nutrition Information

Carbohydrates: 5.5g	Calories: 396
Fat: 21.6g	Sugar: 1.7g
Protein: 44.4g	Fiber: 1.3g

Dinner *Cauliflower Pizza*

Crust:	Topping:
• 1 small head cauliflower (58)	• ¼ cup pizza sauce (40)
*or 2 cups pre-riced	• ⅓ cup red onion, finely chopped (6)
• ½ tsp basil (1)	• 20g cervelat salami (74)
• ¼ tsp garlic powder (2)	• ½ cup light, shredded, tex mex cheese (120)
• ¼ tsp oregano (1)	
• 2 tbsp light mozzarella shredded cheese (29)	• ⅓ bell pepper, green, thinly sliced (4)
• 2 tbsp light grated parmesan cheese (45)	• 5 small white mushrooms, sliced (11)
• 2 tbsp egg whites (15)	

Directions

1. *Preheat oven to 475 degrees fahrenheit*
2. *Rice cauliflower in a blender or food processor*
   to save on time, buy pre riced cauliflower
3. *Put riced cauliflower into bowl, covered with a paper towel, and microwave for 2-3 minutes*
4. *Pour cauliflower onto clean tea towel. cover and twist the towel, removing as much water from the cauliflower as possible*

5. *Put cauliflower back into bowl. add egg, basil, oregano, garlic, parmesan and mozzarella. mix into dough*

6. *Roll out dough into thin circle on parchment paper and carefully put onto oil-sprayed pizza pan (parchment side up).*

7. *Slowly and carefully remove parchment paper*

8. *Baked until edges start to golden*

   *a bit longer for a crispier crust

9. *Remove from oven and add toppings*

10. *Bake again until cheese has melted*

Nutrition Information

Carbohydrates: 27g	Calories: 405
Fat: 8g	Sugar: 13g
Protein: 35g	Fiber: 8g

Exercise

Cardio and Strength: Full body circuit

Minutes	Movement
(0-5)	Warm-up 5 minute jog
(5-40)	3 times through *future attempts • 100 Skips • 90 Arm circles (45 forward, 45 backward) • 80 Resistant punches • 70 Medicine ball russian twists • 60 Mountain climbers • 50 Jumping jacks • 40 Banded squats • 30 Kettlebell swings • 20 Box jumps • 10 Roll outs

	time:_____ *time:_____ *time:_____ time:_____ *time:_____ *time:_____ time:_____ *time:_____ *time:_____

	Stretch
	    chest, shoulders, hip flexors, glute muscles, quads,
	    calves

	Equipment needed skipping rope, resistance band, kettlebell, bench

Day 7

"Let the new adventures begin" —Unkown

Write 3 activities you would enjoy doing with friends and family that doesn't revolve around calories. (List of calorie-free activities on page 85)

1. _____

2. _____

3. _____

Breakfast *Peanut Butter Banana Protein Smoothie*

Ingredients

• ½ banana (52) *peel, slice and freeze bananas when starting to brown for smoothies • 3 tbsp quick oats (56)	• 1 scoop vanilla whey protein isolate (115) • 2 tbsp natural peanut butter (180) • ice & water

Nutrition Information

Carbohydrates: 31g	Calories: 404
Fat: 15g	Sugar: 10g
Protein: 37g	Fiber: 6g

Lunch *Ham Avocado Wrap*

Ingredients

• 6 slices extra lean ham (140) *low sodium ham* • whole grain (180)	• ½ small avocado (80) • 1 tbsp mustard • 1 cup Spinach (7)

Nutrition Information

Carbohydrates: 38g	Calories: 407
Fat: 14g	Sugar: 6g
Protein: 29g	Fiber: 8g

Dinner *Turkey Spaghetti Squash*

• ¾ cup Ground Turkey, extra lean, raw (198)	• ½ cup Pasta Sauce (45)
• 3 cup spaghetti squash (93)	• 5 mushroom, small, white (11)
• 1 tbsp grated parmesan cheese (25)	• 1 tsp red chili flakes (5)
• spices cumin, chili powder, red chili flakes, onion powder, garlic	• 1 clove garlic (4)
	• ¼ cup chopped carrots (12)
	• ½ cup chopped red onion (8)

Directions

1. *Preheat oven to 350 degrees fahrenheit*
2. *Brown turkey slightly on medium sized pan. Add garlic and chopped carrots, onion & mushrooms.*
   1. **optional: add cumin, chili powder, red chili flakes, onion powder and garlic*
3. *Add spaghetti sauce, reduce temperature to low and cover.*
4. *Stab spaghetti squash with fork multiple times and place in the oven. Cooked for 45 minutes -1 hour until slightly soft.*
5. *Once squash is finished, cut in half, remove seeds and scoop out flesh onto a plate. Top with meat sauce and parmesan cheese*

Nutrition Information

Carbohydrates: 37g	Calories: 402
Fat: 15g	Sugar: 18g
Protein: 37g	Fiber: 8g

Exercise

Active Rest Day

Minutes	Movement
(0-40)	Activity: _____

Day 8

"Happiness comes to those who appreciate what they already have"
— Unknown

Name 3 things about your body that you love:

1. _____

2. _____

3. _____

Breakfast _____

Ingredients

• • • •	• • • •

Directions

_____

_____

_____

Nutrition Information

Carbohydrates: _____g Fat: _____g Protein: _____g	Calories: _____ Sugar: _____g Fiber: _____g

Lunch _____

Ingredients

• • • •	• • • •

Directions

_____

_____

_____

Nutrition Information

Carbohydrates: _____g	Calories: _____
Fat: _____g	Sugar: _____g
Protein: _____g	Fiber: _____g

Dinner _____

Ingredients

•	•
•	•
•	•
•	•

Directions

_____

_____

_____

Nutrition Information

Carbohydrates: _____g	Calories: _____
Fat: _____g	Sugar: _____g
Protein: _____g	Fiber: _____g

Exercise

Cardio: High Intensity Interval Training

Minutes	Movement
(0-3)	Warm-up 60 high knees, 50 butt kicks, 40 calf sweeps, 30 backward hip circles, 20 standing glute presses, 10 forward hip circles
(3-29)	Intervals: 4 x [600m Interval Run,30 sec break] *future attempts time:_____ *time:_____ *time:_____ time:_____ *time:_____ *time:_____ time:_____ *time:_____ *time:_____ time:_____ *time:_____ *time:_____
(29-40)	Intervals: 1x [Sprint Set] • 90 seconds fast run • 90 seconds easy jog or walk • 60 seconds fast run • 60 seconds easy jog or walk • 30 seconds fast run • 30 seconds easy jog or walk • 60 seconds fast run • 60 seconds easy jog or walk • 90 seconds fast run • 90 seconds easy jog or walk
	Cool Down and Stretch glute muscles, quads, hip flexors, hamstrings, calves
	Equipment Needed treadmill or outdoor space

Day 9

"Focus on the solution, not the problem" —Jim Rohn

Rather than think about old habits you're trying to break, think about 3 new habits you can begin

    1. _____

    2. _____

    3. _____

Breakfast *Starbucks*

* dining out subjects you to higher than normal sodium intake

Ingredients

• Spinach, Egg white and Feta Wrap (290)	• Tall Skim Milk latte (100)

Nutrition Information

Carbohydrates: 48g	Calories: 390
Fat: 10g	Sugar: 18g
Protein: 29g	Fiber: 6g

Lunch *McDonald's Sandwich*

Option 1: Tomato & Mozzarella w/grilled chicken

no creamy tomato and herb sauce

Nutrition Information

Carbohydrates: 39g	Calories: 390
Fat: 11g	Sugar: 6g
Protein: 35g	Fiber: 3g

Option 2: McDouble Burger

Nutrition Information

Carbohydrates: 34g	Calories: 370
Fat: 17g	Sugar: 7g
Protein: 21g	Fiber: 2g

Option 3: Double Cheeseburger

Nutrition Information

Carbohydrates: 35g	Calories: 420
Fat: 20g	Sugar: 7g
Protein: 24g	Fiber: 2g

a double quarter pounder with cheese has 740 calories and 43g of fat

Dinner *Sushi Dinner*

• 4 pieces (4 oz) tuna sashimi (124) • 3 pieces (3 oz) salmon sashimi (123) • 1 cucumber maki roll (6 pieces) (136)	• 1 tbsp low sodium soy sauce (10) • 2 tbsp pickled ginger (5) • ½ tsp wasabi (8)

Nutrition Information

Carbohydrates: 33g	Calories: 406
Fat: 6g	Sugar: 1g
Protein: 52g	Fiber: 4g

Exercise

Strength Training: Back *Supersets*

Supersets are combinations of exercises performed consecutively without rest in between the sets

Recommended Warm Up: 500 skips

Minutes	Movement		
(0-10)	Superset 1 x 3 sets • 20 kneeling plank rows *w/knees 1 inch off the ground • 20 walkout w/ push up		
(10-20)	Superset 2 x 3 sets • 20 plank row with reverse fly • 20 serratus anterior dips		
(20-30)	Superset 3 x 3 sets • 20 single arm cable rows in lunge position: LEFT • 20 single arm cable rows in lunge position: RIGHT		
(30-40)	Superset 4 x 3 sets • 1 pull up negative • 30 seconds break		
	Stretch back, abs, quads, hamstrings, glute muscles		
	Equipment needed dumbbells, resistance band, cable machine, pull up machine		

Day 10

"Success is not a big step in the future, success is a small step taken right now" — Unknown

When life gets busy and things don't go as planned, what is one small commitment you can make today, no matter what, towards your fitness goals? It can take a little as 5 minutes:

_____

_____

_____

Breakfast *Bagel with Salmon Lox*

Ingredients

• 12 grain bagel (230)	• 1 tbsp capers (2)
• 2 tbsp light herb and garlic cream cheese (60)	• ½ tsp dill (1)
• 3 oz smoked salmon lox (99)	

Nutrition Information

• Carbohydrates: 41g	• Calories: 393
• Fat: 13g	• Sugar: 3g
• Protein: 28g	• Fiber: 5g

Lunch *Greek Zoodle Salad*

Ingredients

• 1 medium zucchini, (made to noodles with spiralizer) (32)	• ¼cup chopped red onion (4)
	• ½ cucumber, sliced (22)
• 2 tbsp light feta and oregano vinaigrette (60)	• 1 tbsp feta cheese (45)

• 1 medium bell pepper, chopped (18) • 5 grape tomatoes, halved (20)	• 4 oz marinated chicken, cubed (187) *½ lemon juice pepper to taste

Nutrition Information

Carbohydrates: 28g Fat: 14g Protein: 47g	Calories: 388 Sugar: 14g Fiber: 4g

Dinner *Chicken and Rice*

• 4oz Skinless Chicken Breast (187) • ½ cup Cooked Brown Rice (109) *with 1 tsp butter (34)	• 10 medium brussel sprouts (75) *steamed with lemon and pepper

Nutrition Information

Carbohydrates: 36g Fat: 9g Protein: 42g	Calories: 405 Sugar: 3g Fiber: 7g

Exercise

Strength and Balance: Lower Body

Minutes	Movement		
(0-4)	Warmup: 1 minute each 1. Jumping jacks 2. Forward jacks 3. Squats (hands out) 4. Slow mountain climbers (foot to outside of hand)		
(4-10)	1. Single Leg Squat 3 sets x10 reps (total sets: 6)		
(10-16)	2. SuperSet • 3 sets x 15 reps squat hops (hands out in front) • 3 sets x 20 reps standing kick-backs (alternate legs: 10 reps each)		
(16-21)	3. Hip Hikes 3 sets x 20 reps (total sets: 6)		
(21-26)	4. Feet-together Glute Thrust 3 sets x 20 reps		
(26-32)	5. Single Leg Deadlift 3 sets x10 reps (total sets: 6)		
(32-40)	6. Lying Leg Lift 3 sets x 15 reps (total sets: 6)		
	Stretch glute muscles, hip flexors, calves, hamstrings, quads		
	Equipment needed barbell, resistance band, bench		

Day 11

"It's not happy people who are grateful, it's grateful people who are happy" —Unknown

Name 3 things you're grateful for that you already have.

1. _____
2. _____
3. _____

Breakfast *Overnight Raspberry Oats*

Ingredients

• ⅓ cup quick oats (120)	• 2 tbsp sliced almonds (122)
• ½ scoop whey protein isolate (58)	• ⅓ cup unsweetened raspberries, fresh or frozen (22)
• 1 tsp chia seed (20)	• ½ cup 0% greek yogurt (67)

Directions

1. *Night before, mix protein powder in ¼ - ½ cup of water to get a very thick liquid in a small container.*
2. *Add oats, almonds and chia seeds, stir*
3. *Top with raspberries. cover and let sit overnight.*
4. *In morning, top with ½ cup 0% greek yogurt and stir.*

Nutrition Information

Carbohydrates: 37g	Calories: 408
Fat: 13g	Sugar: 7g
Protein: 36g	Fiber: 11g

Lunch *Turkey chili*

Ingredients

• 200g (1 heaping cup) raw extra lean ground turkey (280)	• ½ cup pasta sauce (50)
• ⅓ cup chopped zucchini (7)	• ⅓ cup chopped carrots (16)
• 3-4 small white mushrooms, chopped (8)	• 1 medium stalk celery, chopped (6)
• ¼ large bell pepper, any colour, chopped (20)	• 1 ½ cup, red onion, chopped (23)
• 1 large garlic clove (6)	• ½ tsp crushed red pepper flakes

Directions

1. *Brown turkey on frying pan. Remove before fully cooked*
2. *Put all ingredients in a pot or slow cooker and let simmer for minimum 1 hr*

Nutrition Information

Carbohydrates: 25g	Calories: 416
Fat: 16g	Sugar: 12g
Protein: 46g	Fiber: 6g

Dinner *Chicken Quesadilla*

Ingredients

• ½ medium bell pepper, green (12)	seasoning:
• ½ medium bell pepper, red (18)	• 1 tsp chili powder (7)
• ¼ cup chopped red onion (4)	• ½ tsp paprika (3)
• 3 oz raw chicken breast, boneless, skinless (102)	• ¼ tsp onion powder (2)
• ⅓ cup light tex mex shredded cheese (80)	• ¼ tsp garlic powder (2)
	• ¼ tsp cumin (2)
• 1 flax tortilla (170)	• pinch chili flakes (0)

Nutrition Information

Carbohydrates: 36g	Calories: 403
Fat: 13g	Sugar: 6g
Protein: 34g	Fiber: 9g

Exercise

Strength Training: Shoulders and Triceps

Recommended warm-up: 5 minute elliptical

Minutes	Exercise	Notes	Notes
(0-5)	1. Barbell Shoulder Press 3 sets x15 reps		
(5-10)	2. Dumbbell Lateral Delt Raises with twist 3 sets X 15 reps		
(10-15)	3. Bent-over-knee Single Arm Rear Delt Raises 3 sets X 15 reps (total sets: 6)		
(15-20)	4. Front Raises with Plate 3 sets X 15 reps		
(20-25)	5. Tricep Cable Pressdowns 3 sets X 15 reps		
(25-30)	6. Tricep Cable pulldowns 3 sets X 15 reps		
(30-35)	7. Bent-over-bench Tricep Extensions 3 sets x15 reps each (total sets: 6)		
(35-40)	8. Assisted Tricep Dips 3 sets X 15 reps		

	Stretch triceps, shoulders, chest		

	Equipment needed
	    cable machine, bench, dumbbells,
	    plate		

Day 12

> *"Do the best you can until you know better. Then when you know better, do better"* — *Maya Angelo*

It's surprising how many calories restaurants hide into what seem like healthy options. Go online and get to know the nutritional facts of a restaurant you go to often. Decide on one or two healthy options before the next time you go there.

1. _____

_____

2. _____

_____

Breakfast _____

Ingredients

•	•
•	•
•	•
•	•

Directions

_____

_____

_____

Nutrition Information

Carbohydrates: _____g	Calories: _____
Fat: _____g	Sugar: _____g
Protein: _____g	Fiber: _____g

Lunch _____

Ingredients

<ul><li></li><li></li><li></li><li></li></ul>

Directions

_____

_____

_____

Nutrition Information

Carbohydrates: _____g	Calories: _____
Fat: _____g	Sugar:_____g
Protein: _____g	Fiber: _____g

Dinner _____

Ingredients

<ul><li></li><li></li><li></li><li></li></ul>

Directions

_____

_____

_____

Nutrition Information

Carbohydrates: _____g	Calories: _____
Fat: _____g	Sugar: _____g
Protein: _____g	Fiber: _____g

Exercise

Cardio: Circuit Training and Abs

Minutes	Movement
(0-15)	1 minute each, 5 times through • Monster Walks • Squats • Burpees
(15-40)	1 minute each, 5 times through • Twisting Plank • Reverse Crunches • Jack Knives • Double Crunches • Plank (with opposite leg opposite arm raises)
	Stretch lower back, abs
	Equipment needed none

Day 13

"Self control is knowing you can but deciding you won't" — *Unknown*

Think about 3 reasons why you want to eat healthy:

1. _____

2. _____

3. _____

Breakfast *Tim Hortons Breakfast*

*dining out subjects you to high sodium

Option 1: Regular Turkey Bacon Club (400)

Nutrition Information

Carbohydrates: 52g	Calories: 400
Fat: 11g	Sugar: 5g
Protein: 26g	Fiber: 5g

Option 2: Breakfast Sandwich and Latte (410)
- Turkey Sausage Breakfast Sandwich (330)
- Small Latte, unsweetened (80)

Nutrition Information

Carbohydrates: 42g	Calories: 410
Fat: 14g	Sugar: 15g
Protein: 28g	Fiber: 1g

Option 3: Grilled Steak and Egg Breakfast Sandwich (400)

Nutrition Information

Carbohydrates: 34g	Calories: 400
Fat: 20g	Sugar: 4g
Protein: 22g	Fiber: 2g

Option 4: Yogurt and Latte (380)

*caution: high in sugar

- Vanilla Greek Yogurt w/Berries and Almond Granola 198g (270)
- Medium latte, unsweetened (110)

Nutrition Information

Carbohydrates: 55g	Calories: 380
Fat: 5g	Sugar: 25g
Protein: 25g	Fiber: 3g

Lunch *Spicy Turkey Lettuce Wraps*

Ingredients

• 200g (1 heaping cup) lean ground turkey, raw (282) • ½ medium bell pepper, green (14) • ½ medium avocado (100) • spices: cumin, chili flakes, chili powder, garlic	• 1 tbsp sriracha hot sauce (2) • ½ tsp stevia, or other sweetener (0) • 1 tbsp soy sauce, low sodium (5) • ½ head iceberg lettuce (8) • *remove smaller inside leaves

Directions

1. *Mix hot sauce, soy sauce and stevia in small dish*
2. *Brown ground turkey over medium frying pan with spices.*
3. *Add bell peppers and cook until they soften and turkey is no longer pink*
4. *Mash avocado and smooth spoonful over piece of lettuce, top with turkey and pepper*
5. *Top with sriracha soy sauce*

Nutrition Information

Carbohydrates: 12g	Calories: 416
Fat: 23g	Sugar: 1g
Protein: 41g	Fiber: 8g

Dinner *Steak and Mushrooms*

Ingredients

• 6oz top sirloin, raw (315) *with meat higher in fat, calories vary depending on brand and cut • montreal steak spice (0) • 1 tbsp horseradish (15)	• 6 small mushrooms, sliced, sauteed (12) • 1 tsp butter (34) • ¼ cup onion, sliced, white (12) • 8 spears asparagus (26)

Nutrition Information

Carbohydrates: 16g Fat: 22g Protein: 40g	Calories: 405 Sugar: 4g Fiber: 6g

Exercise

Strength and Cardio: Full Body Circuit

Recommended: 5 minute warm-up jog

Minutes	Movement
(0-40)	4 times through: *future attempts 100 High Knees 90 Star calf poppers: 30 Left - 30 Right - 30 Left & Right 80 Water Bottle Toe Taps 70 Plank Twists 60 Walking Lunges 50 3-shuffle Side Lunge w/ Ankle Tap 40 Jump Squats 30 Burpees 20 Tuck Jumps 10 Push Ups 01 minute break

	time:_____ *time:_____ *time:_____ time:_____ *time:_____ *time:_____ time:_____ *time:_____ *time:_____ time:_____ *time:_____ *time:_____

	Stretch
	    hip flexors, calves, abs, quads, ham strings, glute
	    muscles

	Equipment needed none

Day 14

"Don't wait until you've reached your goal to be proud of yourself. Be proud of every step you take towards reaching that goal" — Unknown

Decide on a non-edible reward for yourself once you've completed a small step towards your fitness and health goals.

Small step: _____

Reward: _____

Breakfast *Hiker's Bar (makes 4)*

Ingredients

• ⅓ cup pumpkin seeds (180)	• ½ tsp vanilla extract (6)
• ¼ cup dried cherries (130)	• ¼ cup sunflower seeds (204)
• 1 cup large flake oats (330)	• ¼ cup chopped walnuts (180)
• ½ tsp cinnamon (3)	• ¼ cup sliced almonds (190)
• 1 ½ bananas (158)	• 2 tbsp hemp hearts (114)

Directions

1. *Preheat oven to 350 degrees fahrenheit*
2. *Grease small baking tray and line with parchment paper (leaving overhang)*
3. *Mash banana until smooth*
4. *Stir in vanilla*
5. *Blend oats until coarsely chopped and add to banana mix*
6. *Stir in hemp hearts, almonds, walnuts, pumpkin seeds, sunflower seeds, cherries and cinnamon*
7. *Wet hands and transfer dough to parchment lined tray. compact down and spread until even*
8. *Bake around 15 minutes until starting to golden around the edges*
9. *Let cool and gently remove from tray to cool.*
10. *Slice into 4 equal parts*

    * freeze remaining

Nutrition Information/per bar

Carbohydrates: 38.5g	Calories: 389
Fat: 21.5g	Sugar: 12.5g
Protein: 13g	Fiber: 6g

Lunch *Cheese and Crackers*

Ingredients

• 20 high fibre crackers (216)	• 45g cheddar cheese (180) *depending on size, ~3 thin slices

Nutrition Information

Carbohydrates: 40g	Calories: 396
Fat: 20g	Sugar: 4g
Protein: 16g	Fiber: 9g

Dinner *Wing-Style Chicken*

Ingredients

• 6 oz chicken thigh, boneless, skinless, raw (195)	• ¼ tsp cayenne (1)
• ¼ cup all-purpose flour (110)	• ¼ cup hot sauce (0) * high in sodium
• 1 tbsp butter (102)	• 1 tsp garlic
• ¼ tsp paprika (2)	• ¼ tsp black pepper

Directions

1. *Mix cayenne, paprika and flour in a small bowl*
2. *Cut chicken into thin strips and place in a large bowl, cover with flour. Mix until well coated. Put in fridge for 1-2 hours uncovered*
3. *Preheat oven to 425 degrees fahrenheit*

4. *Bake until no longer pink*
   about 10-12 minutes
5. *Melt butter in large microwave safe bowl*
   about 10-15 seconds
6. *Add hot sauce, pepper and garlic. Mix well*
7. *Add chicken strips, mix until well coated and serve*

Nutrition Information

Carbohydrates: 25g	Calories: 419
Fat: 19g	Sugar: 0g
Protein: 37g	Fiber: 2g

*1 lb of restaurant-style wings is roughly 900-1100 calories and approximately 50g fat

Exercise

Active Rest Day

Minutes	Movement
(0-40)	Activity: _____

Day 15

"Once you control your mind, you can conquer your body" — Unknown

T - H - I - N - K about your thoughts.

Is what you're thinking TRUE? Is it HELPFUL to think this way? Are your thoughts INSPIRING you? Are your thoughts NECESSARY? Are you being KIND to yourself?

Create a thought that meets all of these criteria:

_____

_____

_____

Breakfast *Banana Peanut Butter Protein Pancake*

Ingredients

• ¼ cup 1% cottage cheese (50) • ½ cup egg whites (60) • ½ scoop whey isolate protein powder (58) • ¼ cup uncooked oats (90)	• 1 tbsp natural peanut butter (90) • ½ small banana (44) • ½ tsp Cinnamon (3) • ¼ tsp Baking powder (0)

Directions

1. *Blend oats into flour*
2. *Add egg whites, protein powder, cottage cheese, peanut butter, banana, cinnamon and baking powder*
3. *Spray frying pan over medium heat*
4. *Pour batter onto pan*
5. *Flip when bubbles form*

Nutrition Information

Carbohydrates: 36g Fat: 10g Protein: 43g	Calories: 395 Sugar: 11g Fiber: 6g

Lunch *Prawn Goat Cheese Salad*

Ingredients

• 3 oz spinach (20)
• 4 oz marinated prawns, peeled (79)
    2 tbsp lemon juice (6)
    pepper to taste
• 2 tbsp walnuts, chopped (100)
• 3 tbsp goat cheese (75)
• ¼ cup dried cranberries, unsweetened (30)
	• dressing:
	• 1 tbsp lemon juice (3)
	• ½ tbsp olive oil (60)
	• 1 tsp maple syrup (18)
	• 1 tsp honey dijon mustard (5)
	• pepper to taste

Nutrition Information

Carbohydrates: 23g Fat: 23g Protein: 28g	Calories: 396 Sugar: 9g Fiber: 6g

Dinner *Steak Skewers and Zucchini Boats*

Steak skewers	Zucchini boats
• 4 oz grilling steak, cubed (180) • ½ tbsp extra virgin olive oil (59) • montreal steak spice (0) • ½ bell pepper, any color (10)	• 1 medium zucchini, split in half (32) • 2 tbsp sun-dried tomatoes (35) • 2 tbsp feta cheese (90) • salt, pepper and basil, to taste

Nutrition Information

Carbohydrates: 16g Fat: 24g Protein: 35g	Calories: 406 Sugar: 6g Fiber: 4g

Exercise

Cardio: Calorie based

Minutes	Movement
(0-5)	Warm-up 5 minutes easy pace elliptical
(5-40)	How fast can you burn 400 calories on elliptical? *future attempts time: _____ *time: _____ *time: _____
	Stretch pecs, biceps, triceps, back, glutes, hamstring, calves, quads
	Equipment needed Elliptical machine

Day 16

"Always have a backup plan" —Mila Kunis

Have a backup, healthy meal option. Whether it be a drive through go-to or a microwave dish you keep in the cupboard or freezer. Avoid being rushed and making impulsive decisions.

_____

_____

_____

Breakfast _____

Ingredients

•	•
•	•
•	•
•	•

Directions

_____

_____

_____

Nutrition Information

Carbohydrates: _____g	Calories: _____
Fat: _____g	Sugar: _____g
Protein: _____g	Fiber: _____g

Lunch _____

Ingredients

•	•
•	•
•	•
•	•

Directions

_____

_____

_____

Nutrition Information

Carbohydrates: _____g	Calories: _____
Fat: _____g	Sugar: _____g
Protein: _____g	Fiber: _____g

Dinner _____

Ingredients

• • • •	• • •

Directions

_____

_____

_____

Nutrition Information

Carbohydrates: _____g	Calories: _____
Fat: _____g	Sugar: _____g
Protein: _____g	Fiber: _____g

Exercise

Strength Training: Back

Recommended warm-up: 5 minutes elliptical

Minutes	Movement	Notes	Notes
(0-5)	1. Dumbbell Pullovers 3 sets x15 reps		
(5-15)	2. 1-Arm Cable Pressdowns 3 sets x 15 reps (total sets: 6)		
(15-20)	3. Seated Cable row Reverse flies 3 sets x 20 reps		
(20-25)	4. Front Raise '21s' 3 sets x 21 reps		
(25-30)	5. Narrow Grip pull ups 3 sets x 10 reps		
(30-35)	6. Resistance Band Posture Holds 3 sets x 30 seconds		
(35-40)	7. Plank Dumbbell Rows 3 sets x 30 reps (15 reps each)		
	Stretch back, biceps, triceps		
	Equipment needed dumbbells, resistance band, pull up machine, cable machine		

Day 17

"Extremes are easy. Strive for balance." — *Colin Wright*

Fill in option C with a balanced approach to each situation.

1. After an unhealthy breakfast and lunch:

   a. Continue with an unhealthy dinner and start fresh tomorrow.

   b. Not eat dinner as punishment for such an unhealthy day.

   c. _____

   _____

   _____

2. After missing Monday, Tuesday, and Wednesday's workouts, deciding on Thursday to:

   a. Write off the rest of the week and aim to workout every day starting Monday.

   b. Work out twice a day for the remainder of the week and drastically decrease food intake to compensate.

   c. _____

   _____

   _____

3. After eating a handful of candy or popcorn from a very large bag:

   a. Decide to eat the entire bag because "who cares, the damage is already done".

   b. Criticize and judge yourself for your idea of a *'lack of self control.'*

   c. _____

   _____

   _____

Breakfast *Pumpkin Pie Smoothie*

Ingredients

• 1 scoop Vanilla Protein (115)	• 2 tsp. cinnamon (11)
• ½ cup 1% cottage cheese (100)	• 1 tsp. ground cloves (6)
• 1 tbsp fiber blend (70)	• 1 tsp. ground allspice (5)
• 2/3 cup canned pumpkin (42)	• 1 tbsp. walnuts (63)

Nutrition Information

Carbohydrates: 34g	Calories: 412
Fat: 13g	Sugar: 11g
Protein: 49g	Fiber: 16g

Lunch *Subway Sandwich*

Ingredients

• 6 inch sweet onion chicken teriyaki (290) • 9 grain wheat • cheddar (60)	• red onion, lettuce, tomato, green pepper, cucumber (10) • avocado (60) • no sauce

Nutrition Information

Carbohydrates: 48g	Calories: 420
Fat: 14g	Sugar: 7g
Protein: 30g	Fiber: 7g

Dinner *Salmon and Beets*

• 4oz salmon, farmed, baked (235) • 1 tbsp chopped walnuts (48)	• 2 medium beets (2" diameter) (71) • 2 tbsp goat cheese (50)

Nutrition Information

Carbohydrates: 18g	Calories: 403
Fat: 23g	Sugar: 12g
Protein: 32g	Fiber: 5g

Exercise

High Intensity: Lower Body with Plyo Intervals

Minutes	Movement	Notes	Notes
(0-2)	Warm up 10 bodyweight squats 10 forward hip circles (5 Left, 5 Right) 10 backward hip circles (5 Left, 5 Right) 10 kickbacks (5 Left, 5 Right)		
(2-5)	Timed Superset: 3 x no break [30 jumping jacks, 10 burpees] time: _____		
(5-13)	Superset 1: 3 sets • 10 Weighted Lunges: Left • 20 Pulse Lunges: Left • 10 Weighted Lunges: Right • 20 Pulse Lunges: Right		
(13-20)	Superset 2: 3 sets • 10 Kettlebell Banded Sumo Squats • 20 Banded Hop Squats		
(20-26)	Superset 3: 3 sets • 30 seconds Medicine Ball Wall Sit • 10 Laying Swiss Ball Kickdowns		
(26-35)	Superset 4: 3 sets • 10 Weighted Curtsy Lunges: Left • 20 Side Step-Ups: Left • 10 Weighted Curtsy Lunges: Right • 20 Side Step-ups: Left		

(35-40)	Timed Superset: 3 x no break [30 jumping jacks, 10 burpees] time:_____ *match or beat initial attempt		

	Stretch
	    glute muscles, calves, hamstrings,
	    quads, abs, lower back		

	Equipment needed
	    dumbbells, kettlebell, resistance
	    band, medicine ball, swiss ball		

Day 18

*"The sexiest thing in the entire world is being really smart.
And being thoughtful. And being generous. Everything
else is crap"* — Ashton Kutcher

What are 3 qualities you pride yourself in that have nothing to do with appearance?

1. _____

2. _____

3. _____

Breakfast *Cheerios and Protein Yogurt*

Ingredients

• 1 cup 0% Greek Yogurt (133) • ½ scoop Vanilla whey isolate protein powder (58)	• 1 cup cheerios (100) • 2 tbsp chopped peanuts (112)

Directions

Mix protein powder and yogurt before adding nuts or cheerios

Nutrition Information

Carbohydrates: 32g Fat: 12g Protein: 45g	Calories: 403 Sugar: 9g Fiber: 7g

Lunch *Tuna Sandwich*

Ingredients

• 1 can tuna (120) • ⅓ cup 0% greek yogurt (43) • 1 tbsp capers, drained (2)	• 1 tsp dijon mustard (5) • ½ tbsp dill (4) • 2 slices 12 grain bread (240) *toasted*

Directions

Mix tuna and yogurt thoroughly. Add capers, dill,and mustard.
*add salt and pepper to taste

Nutrition Information

Carbohydrates: 43g	Calories: 414
Fat: 5g	Sugar: 8g
Protein: 46g	Fiber: 6g

Dinner *Shepherd's Pie (4 servings)*
*freeze leftovers

Ingredients

• 450g (2 ¼ cup raw) extra lean ground turkey (585)	• 1 tbsp olive oil (120)
• 9 cups (2 medium heads) cauliflower (232)	• 1 tbsp au jus gravy mix (20)
	• ½ tbsp parsley (2)
• 4 cloves garlic (16)	• 1 tbsp ketchup (20)
• 1 cup diced red onion (16)	• 2 tbsp butter (203)
• 5 medium celery stalks (32)	• 1 cup light shredded cheese (240)
• 3 medium carrots (82)	• pepper to taste

Directions

1. *Preheat oven 400 degrees fahrenheit*
2. *Boil or steam chopped cauliflower until soft. Drain and set aside to cool*
   *can buy pre-riced cauliflower to save time
3. *Heat olive oil, garlic, onion, celery and carrot in medium size frying pan for 3-5 minutes*
4. *Add ground turkey and cook until still slightly pink*
5. *Add gravy mix to 1/2 cup warm water until dissolved. Add gravy to turkey and vegetables.*

6. *Add parsley, ketchup and pepper. Cover and simmer.*
7. *Blend cauliflower until smooth.*
8. *Mix in butter until melted*
9. *Pour turkey and vegetable mixture into lightly greased casserole dish. Spread into even layer.*
10. *Add cauliflower to casserole dish to form a second later. Smooth with a spoon*
11. *Top with cheese and bake until cheese is melted and edges are golden*

Nutrition Information/serving

Carbohydrates: 24g	Calories: 392
Fat: 22g	Sugar: 4g
Protein: 32g	Fiber: 10.5g

Exercise

High Intensity Strength Training: Upper Body

Minutes	Movement	Notes	Notes
(0-2)	Warm-up 20 Arm Circles (forward) 20 Arm Circles (backward) 20 Jumping Jacks		
(2-5)	Timed Superset: 3 x through, no breaks • 10 left arm Pushup • 10 right arm Pushup • 10 Pushups time: _____		

(5-13)	Superset 1 x 4 sets • 10 heavy dumbbell Shoulder Press • 20 light Dumbbell Alternating Shoulder Press		
(13-21)	Superset 2 x 4 sets • 10 Dumbbell Tricep Extension • 20 Tricep Bench Dips		
(21-29)	Superset 3 x 4 sets • 10 front (anterior) delt raises • 40 resistance band punches		
(29-37)	Superset 4 x 4 sets • 10 rear delt High Pulls • 20 rear delt L-Lifts		
(37-30)	Timed Superset: 3 x through, no breaks • 10 left arm Pushup • 10 right arm Pushup • 10 Pushups time: _____ *match or beat initial attempt		
	Stretch 　　chest, shoulders, triceps		
	Equipment needed 　　dumbbells, resistance band, bench		

Day 19

"Whatever's good for your soul. Do that" — Unknown

Find 1 new quote that inspires you. Write it down and stick it on your wall.

_____

_____

_____

Breakfast *Pumpkin Chai Breakfast Granola*

Ingredients

• ⅓ cup pumpkin puree (20) • ¼ tbsp cinnamon (1) • ¼ tsp nutmeg (2) • 1 tsp pure vanilla extract (12)	• ¾ cup 2% plain greek yogurt (120) • 4-5 drops liquid stevia (0) • 1 tsp pre-made Chai spice* (24) *sugar, cardamom, ginger, cinnamon, nutmeg, pepper* • ⅔ cup Granola cereal (210)

Directions

1. *Mix all ingredients into yogurt except granola. Can leave in fridge overnight.*
2. *Add granola when ready to serve.*

Nutrition Information: per serving

Carbohydrates: 46g Fat: 12g Protein: 22g	Calories: 390 Sugar: 25g Fiber: 7g

Lunch *Pita (from Pita Pit)*

note: dining out is subject to inaccuracy and higher sodium levels

Ingredients

• Small Pita (Petita Wheat) (130) • Cheddar cheese (109) • Double Roast beef (120)	• Alfalfa sprouts, cucumbers, green peppers, jalapenos, iceberg lettuce, onions (15) • Horseradish dijon mustard (34)

Nutrition Information

Carbohydrates: 34g Fat: 18g Protein: 28g	Calories: 408 Sugar: 3g Fiber: 7g

Dinner *Sushi Salad Bowl*

Ingredients

• 2 cups 50/50 spinach and mixed greens (13) • ½ cup daikon (5) • ⅓ cup cooked brown rice (75)	• ½ small tomato, sliced (5) • 4 tbsp horseradish and miso hummus (184) • 4-5 slices (4oz) tuna sashimi (124)

Nutrition Information

Carbohydrates: 38g Fat: 12g Protein: 35g	Calories: 406 Sugar: 5g Fiber: 8.1g

Exercise

Cardio and Strength: Lower Body Circuit

Recommended Warm-up: 5 minute jog

Minutes	Movement		
(0-40)	5 x 1 minute each • Speed Skaters • Around the world lunges • Split lunges • Rocket squats		
	• Step ups: left • Step ups: right • Box squat jacks • Rest		
	Stretch glute muscles, hamstrings, quads		
	Equipment needed box or bench		

Day 20

"Education, more than anything else, improves our chances of building better lives" — Nelson Mandela

Be an informed and educated consumer. Many packaged products are very strategic in their nutrition label. Go into your kitchen and look at 3 products. Research ingredients you don't know and pay attention to what a serving size is.

1. _____

2. _____

3. _____

Nutrition

Breakfast _____

Ingredients

•	•
•	•
•	•
•	•

Directions

_____

_____

_____

Nutrition Information

Carbohydrates: _____g	Calories: _____
Fat: _____g	Sugar: _____g
Protein: _____g	Fiber: _____g

Lunch _____

Ingredients

-
-
-
-

-
-
-
-

Directions

_____

_____

_____

Nutrition Information

Carbohydrates: _____g	Calories: _____
Fat: _____g	Sugar: _____g
Protein: _____g	Fiber: _____g

Dinner _____

Ingredients

-
-
-
-

-
-
-
-

Directions

_____

_____

_____

Nutrition Information

Carbohydrates: _____g	Calories: _____
Fat:_____g	Sugar: _____g
Protein: _____g	Fiber: _____g

Exercise

Cardio: Circuit and Abs

Minutes	Movement		
(0-15)	1 minute each, 5 times through • Butt Kicks • 3-Shuffle Run • Mountain Climbers		
(15-40)	1 minute each, 5 times through • Weight Crunches • Dumbbell Leg Raises • Roman Chair Weighted Obliques • Cable Woodchops • Plank		
	stretch lower back, abs		
	Equipment needed roman chain, dumbbells, cable		

Snack Ideas

<u>Banana & Peanut Butter (195)</u>

Medium Banana (105)
1 tbsp PB (90)

<u>Veggies & Hummus (181)</u>

4 tbsp Hummus (120)
100g Carrot Sticks (41)
100g Bell Pepper (20)

<u>Protein Bar (160-300)</u>
        *look for whole food ingredients

<u>Chips, Salsa and Guacamole (275)</u>

24 Chips (140)
        *look for high fiber, low calorie options

Guacamole Individual Cup (100)

½ Cup Salsa (35)

<u>Butter and Popcorn (202)</u>
high fiber

1 small individual bag, plain (100)
1 tbsp butter (102)
seasoning (0)

<u>Protein Yogurt (248)</u>

¾ cup 0% plain greek yogurt (100)
½ scoop protein powder, any flavour (58)
2 tbsp unsweetened coconut, flaked (90)

<u>Sugar Free Gummy Bears (153)</u>
high fiber

1 pack stevia-sweetened gummies (153)

<u>Daikon (61)</u>
1 medium daikon, fresh, sliced into sticks
sprinkle with lime juice and salt (61)

CALORIE-FREE ACTIVITIES

- Aquarium
- Bowling
- Snowshoeing
- Shopping
- Dance class
- Homeless Shelter volunteering
- Coffee date
- Holiday event
- Scenic walk
- Comedy Show
- Live Music
- Spa: nails, massage, etc.
- Skating
- Movies
- Hair salon
- Thrift store shopping
- Floating tank
- Painting class
- What's on groupon?
- Swimming at the pool
- Yoga
- museum
- Curling
- Tourist in your own city/town
- Hockey Game
- Casino Night
- Chinatown
- Festive Parade
- Trampoline park
- Arcade
- Miniputt
- Local Hike
- Go Karting
- Outdoor movie theatres
- An Escape Room challenge
- Rock climbing
- Wave pool
- Kayaking
- Horseback riding
- Driving range
- Horse track races
- Farmer's market
- Fair
- Drive-In movies
- Water Slides
- Wine tasting on bikes
- Swimming (lake/ocean)
- Camping
- Batting Cages
- Boating
- Bonfire
- Shooting at Gun Range
- BBQ
- Bingo
- Baseball game

CONCLUSION

Losing weight, and then maintaining a desired weight is tough. I know from personal experience. Weight loss and control has always been a focus for me because I've struggled with both for a long time. After all, most of us love to eat, and go out and be social, and such spontaneous activities don't necessarily jibe with consuming controlled portions of food or drink.

What I've learned through my education and subsequent research is that while there is a tremendous amount of information about weight control out there (much of it presented by the multi-billion dollar weight loss industry), good health is largely found through trial and error, and is highly specific to the individual.

I do believe, however, that the most important prerequisite to a successful weight control/health program is to maintain a positive and motivated mindset. If one has that, and then consistently follows a nutritionally healthy diet along with a regular exercise regime, one is bound to succeed .

My goal in writing 'The Mind, the Motion' was to provide what I hope are helpful strategies that will put the reader's mind and body in a healthier place. There will always be days of self-doubt and feelings of defeat; however, the key to success is to quickly get back on track and decrease unhealthy habits. Consistency is critical to making change, and a consistently positive mindset will assist in 'self-doubt' days being eliminated altogether.

Achieving a happier state is the reason most of us seek change, so make sure whatever is taken from this book makes you, the reader just that – Happy. Enjoy the journey. If we aren't creating happier versions of ourselves, what's the point of it all?

ABOUT THE AUTHOR

After receiving a Bachelor of Arts in Psychology from the University of British Columbia, the author spent a number of years researching nutrition and exercise sciences and applying what she learned to her own life. She is a certified personal trainer through the American Council on Exercise, specialized in behaviour change. She is also an Ironman Triathlon finisher, and has competed seven times in the British Columbia Amateur BodyBuilding Association. Finally, she is the founder of Fit2Live Fitness: an online-based personal training company focused on weight control and confidence building.

www.ingramcontent.com/pod-product-compliance
Lightning Source LLC
Chambersburg PA
CBHW070812280326
41934CB00012B/3168